30 Amazing Weight Loss Workouts You Can Do
From The Comfort Of Your Own Home!

John Mayo

TO
SUPER SOPHIE
I HOPE THIS TEACHES
YOU THAT PERSEVERANCE
PAYS OFF.
AND SKIPPING IS WAY
COOLER THAN RUNNING

:)

DAD
xxx

Table of Contents:

Chapter 1: Introduction

Fitness cannot get much more simple than this. All you will need for the workouts in this book is a jump rope. I initially got into using skipping as a fitness tool when I started boxing a few years ago. While I only trained boxing for about 9 months, the fitness techniques I learned during that brief time have enhanced my personal workout program. As you probably know, jump rope is one of the main forms of cardiovascular training in boxing. They don't do this exercise because it's fun (even though it can be); they do it because it's hard as hell and it dramatically increases your foot speed, agility, coordination, endurance and lung capacity.

If you've read some of my other fitness books then you already know that I absolutely love jump rope. I find it very challenging and I feel that you get more out of it in a shorter time when compared to something like jogging. If you jump rope for fifteen minutes as opposed to jogging for fifteen minutes I guarantee you will be more tired when you finish jumping rope. The best part about jumping rope is that the more you do it, the more fun you will have with it. There are lots of advanced skipping moves and workouts that you can do to push yourself as you get better.

I have laid this book out in as simple a format as possible. First, I will discuss the key exercises in the book so that we are all on the same page. Next, I will give you 10 beginner, 10 intermediate and 10 advanced workouts that you can do from the comfort of your own home. These workouts will be fairly detailed and easy to follow. It is suggested that you warm-up before each workout. I advise that you to try to do all 30 of these workouts over the span of 30 days. Keep in mind that if this is your first time skipping you may get very frustrated at the start. I remember my first week of skipping and I dreaded it with a passion. Once you get comfortable with a skipping rope all of the various techniques will fall into place quite quickly. Let's get down to business!

Chapter 2: Explanation of Key Exercises

Here I will be explaining all of the exercises that you will have to do in this book. I will do my best to explain them all but if any of them seem unclear there are certainly YouTube videos out there that can give you a more in-depth idea on how to do particular exercises. This book wouldn't be very fun if the workouts only involved jump rope, so many of the workouts include other body weight exercises.

Understanding Workout Terminology:

When reading a workout the first number is the number of sets and the second number is the number of repetitions per set. So if you see 4 x 20, that means four sets of twenty reps per set. During a set you perform every exercise in order with no rest between exercises unless otherwise instructed. Some workouts will be timed such as 3 x 1:00, 1:00 off, 1:30 on. For this workout you would be doing each exercise in the set for one minute, resting for one minute and then doing that same exercise for one and a half minutes.

Jump Rope:

Make sure the skipping rope is the proper length. You can check this by holding the rope out in front of you, stepping on it with one foot and ensuring that the base of the handles comes up to at least your nipples. You can skip in a stationary position, or you can move around while skipping. Remember your arms should be doing very little work while you are skipping, you should be moving the ropes mostly with your wrists. Try to keep your feet together and stay on your toes. Take small jumps to avoid wasting energy.

Speed Skipping:

The key to speed skipping is to ensure that you are not jumping too high off the ground. Take small hops and let the rope pass under your feet as fast as you possibly can.

Single Leg Skip:

This is just like regular jump rope except for you only use 1 leg at a time.

Double Under:

Each time you jump the rope should pass under your feet twice.

Cross Over's:

Cross your arms in front of you while jumping rope. You should get into a rhythm when doing this kind of skipping. The rhythm should go like this: one jump regular, one jump crossover, one jump regular, one jump crossover (alternate the lead arm each time you crossover).

Jumping Jack Skipping:

While jumping rope open and close your legs while jumping, just like your are doing a jumping jack.

Ski Skipping:

With your feet together and your knees slightly bent, hop from side to side while jumping rope as if you were downhill skiing.

Boxing Jump Rope:

This is hard to master, but once you get it down it becomes fluid and simple. Essentially, while jumping rope you want to bring your right heel to your butt while your left foot jumps regularly. On the next jump you want to kick your right foot out in front of you so that the heel touches the ground while jumping regularly with your left foot. Then you repeat the same motion but with your left foot. You want to alternate legs and go back and fourth so it ends up like this: right foot heel to butt, right foot heel to floor, left foot heel to butt, left foot heel to floor. I know this sounds complicated but it really isn't that bad.

Heel Skipping:

This is very hard to master. You want to make sure you have shoes with good heel support for this one. Basically you want to speed skip but on the heels of your feet. This sounds easier than it is.

Double Under Crossover:

This is probably the hardest skipping move that I can do (but keep in mind I'm no pro. I didn't even include triple or quadruple unders since I don't want to preach what I can't practice myself). For this move you need to perform a double under, but on the second 'under' you need to do a crossover.

Freestyle Skipping:

While freestyle skipping you can essentially do whatever you want. You could start by just doing normal jump rope, then you might do some double unders, single leg skipping, boxing jump rope and heel skipping. It's totally up to you. Challenge yourself while freestyle skipping and try some moves you're not overly comfortable with. You could do 15 reps of each of the skipping exercises listed above for starters.

The Pushup:

Your stomach should be flat on the ground. Keep your arms at shoulder width apart, keep your back straight and make sure your chest touches the ground at the bottom and that your arms are straight at the end of every repetition.

The Burpee:

Start in the standing position, jump down until your chest is on the ground, do a pushup keeping your back flat, jump your legs up into a squatted position and spring yourself up into the air with your arms reaching to the sky. With practice this movement will become fluid, but it will remain a very challenging exercise.

The Squat Jump:

Squats should be performed with your feet at shoulder width apart. Put your arms straight out in front of you and keep your back straight as you lower your bum to your ankles, keeping your legs parallel to one-another. Keep your back straight and keep your weight on your heels. Once you get as low as you can, use your legs to push yourself back up and jump into the air about 1 foot. Make sure to keep your back straight and your core tight. Use the momentum of the squat to get yourself into the air on the jump.

The Mountain Climber:

Mountain climbers are great for your core. To perform, hover above the ground keeping your body horizontal. You should be on your toes and hands with your arms straight. One at a time, bring your knees towards your chest in an alternating motion. Every time both legs go in and out, you have completed one repetition.

The Lunge Walk:

One leg at a time, step one foot out in front of you as far as you can, while dropping the opposite knee down to the ground (don't actually touch the knee on the ground, but get as close as you can). Get a nice smooth walking pattern going as you continue to switch legs.

The Reverse Crunch:

Reverse crunches are performed by lying flat on your back with your hands on the ground beside you. Your legs should be bent with your feet on the ground and you simply bring your knees up towards your chest and then back down to perform one repetition.

Speed Skaters:

Swing your left leg behind you (in a sort of sideways lunge) and touch your right foot with your right hand, then swing your right leg behind you and touch your left foot with your left hand to complete one rep.

Jumping Jacks:

Hop your legs in towards each other and then hop them out until they are past shoulder width. While jumping your straight arms should be simultaneously following the motion of your legs. Essentially when your legs come together, your arms are at your side, when you jump your legs apart your arms swing up towards the sky so that your whole body looks like a star.

Seal Jacks:

This is just like a jumping jack but instead of raising your arms above your head, you clap your hands in front of your face while keeping your arms straight. Your legs should be jumping in and out exactly like they would in a jumping jack.

Wall Sits:

Put your back flat against a wall, bend your legs at about 90 degrees and hover above the ground like you are sitting in an invisible chair. Hold the position for as long as the specified time says.

The Plank:

 For a plank you want your stomach facing the ground. Put your elbows underneath your shoulders and lift yourself off the ground. Your weight should be on your elbows and your toes. Try to keep your back perfectly flat (don't sag your hips down to the ground or lift your bum really high into the air). Keep your abs tight and ensure that you have a comfortable base on your elbows/ forearms.

Chapter 3: 10 Beginner Workouts

(1) 4 Sets of:

- 2:00 jump rope
- 30 seconds speed skipping
- 30 seconds plank
- 20 seconds mountain climbers

*Rest 20 seconds between exercises and 1:30 between sets.

NOTES: This workout will engage your core and test your skipping abilities. If you mess up during a timed skipping exercise in any of the workouts, try to get right back to the exercise as soon as you recover from your mistake.

(2) 4 X 25 reps of the following exercises:

- Single leg skip (right)
- Single leg skip (left)
- Ski Skips
- Crossovers
- Speed skipping

* No rest between exercises. Rest 2 minutes after each set.

NOTES: Try to transition between exercises as fast as possible. Don't waste any time!

(3) Complete 3 sets of the following:

100 jump rope

20 squat jumps

30 mountain climbers

40 jumping jacks

50 jump rope

*Rest 20 seconds between exercises and 2 minutes between sets.

(4) In 8 minutes complete as many sets as you can:

30 speed skipping

5 burpees

15 speed skaters

10 squat jumps

* No designated rest at all during this workout. You're trying to see how many sets you can complete. Try to set a consistent pace and hold it for the entire 15 minutes. Obviously you will have to rest, but you should try to space out this rest time and minimize it as much as possible.

(5) 4 X 20 reps of the following exercises

- Pushups

- Crossovers

- Reverse Crunches
- Ski Skipping
- Seal Jacks
- Speed Skipping
- Mountain Climbers
- Boxing Jump Rope

* Rest 30 seconds between exercises and 2:30 minutes between sets.

NOTES: This workout will test your skipping ability by incorporating many different skipping techniques.

(6) Complete 2 sets of the following:

30 seconds jump rope

30 seconds plank

1:00 jump rope

1:00 plank

1:30 jump rope

1:30 plank

2:00 jump rope

2:00 plank

*No rest between exercises. Rest 3 minutes between sets.

NOTES: If you can't hold the plank for the specified time, simply take a short rest when you need to and then get right back into plank position as soon as you can.

(7) Perform each exercise for 45 seconds, rest for 30 seconds and then perform the same exercise for 30 seconds. Once you do the exercise twice, rest for 1:30 and move down the list. Complete 1 set of the following:

- Speed skipping
- Burpees
- Wall sits
- Single leg skip (left)
- Single leg skip (right)
- Lunge walks
- Freestyle skipping

(8) In 20 minutes do as many jump ropes (or freestlye skipping) as you can. Record the number in a workout journal so that you can do this workout again in the future and track your progress. You may find it difficult to keep count and it's not overly important that you do. The important thing is that you skip for 20 minutes straight. If you make mistakes resume skipping as soon as you can.

(9) 4 X 20 seconds of each exercise:

- Speed skipping
- Mountain climbers
- Ski skipping
- Push-ups
- Boxing jump rope
- Burpees

* Rest 20 seconds between exercises and 1 minute between sets.

NOTES: This workout is meant to be very intense. One set is complete once you do 20 seconds of each exercise. Push yourself as hard as you can during the 20-second pieces and try to do as many reps as you can.

(10) 6 X 30 reps of the following exercises:

- Boxing jump rope
- Single leg skip (right)
- Single leg skip (left)
- Ski Skips
- Crossovers
- Speed skipping
- Jumping jack skipping

* No rest between exercises. Rest 2 minutes after each set.

NOTES: Try to transition between exercises as fast as possible. Don't waste any time!

Chapter 4: 10 Intermediate Workouts

(1) You have 15 minutes to complete all of the repetitions of the following exercises:

400 jump rope

30 burpees

60 push-ups

100 reverse crunches

50 lunge walks

100 double unders

*Rest as you need, but try to get it all done in 15 minutes.

NOTES: You don't have to go down the list as you would in a normal workout. For example, you could do 100 jump ropes, 10 lunge walks, 5 burpees, 20 push-ups, 30 reverse crunches, etc. Just make sure that you keep track of your repetitions. You could use a white board or a pen and paper.

(2) 2 X 10 minutes jump rope. Each 10 minutes is broken down as follows:

2:00 jump rope

1:00 speed skipping

30 seconds single leg skip (left leg)

30 seconds single leg skip (right leg)

1:00 ski skipping

1:00 boxing jump rope

30 seconds heel skipping

30 seconds crossovers

2:00 jumping jack skipping

1:00 double unders

*No rest during the 10 minutes. Rest 3 minutes between sets.

(3) Complete 2 sets of the following:

50 double unders, 50 jumping jacks

40 double unders, 40 seal jacks

30 double unders, 30 mountain climbers

20 double unders, 20 reverse crunches

10 double unders, 10 push ups

5 double unders, 5 burpees

*Rest 30 seconds between exercises (meaning that you rest only after the non-skipping exercises. For example, you would do 50 double unders, 50 jumping jacks and then rest for 30 seconds). Rest 3 minutes between sets

NOTES: Do double unders if possible. If you can't do double unders then do speed skipping for double the amount of jumps (Example: if you can't do 50 double unders then do 100 regular jumps as fast as you can).

(4) Complete one set of the following:

5:00 jump rope

50 seconds plank

4:00 freestyle skipping

40 seal jacks

3:00 freestyle skipping

30 lunge walks

2:00 speed skipping

20 squat jumps

1:00 speed skipping

10 push-ups

* Rest 30 seconds between exercises.

(5) Complete as many sets as possible in 10 minutes:

25 double unders

5 squat jumps

3 burpees

*Rest as needed but remember you want to see how many sets you can do. Try to minimize your rest time. For example, you could rest for 20 seconds only after you complete 3 sets.

NOTES: At first glance this workout may not seem like it will be too difficult, but don't fool yourself. I purposely made the sets short so that you have to do a lot of them within the 10-minute period. This workout is sure to burn!

(6) Complete 4 sets of the following exercises:

2:00 freestyle skipping
1:30 plank
25 lunge walks
1:00 wall sit
15 squat jumps
20 double unders

*Rest 30 seconds between exercises and 2:00 between sets

NOTES: This workout is sure to push your legs to the limit!

(7) Complete 1 set of the following:

10 double unders, 1 push-up

9 double unders, 2 push-ups

8 double unders, 3 push-ups

7 double unders, 4 push-ups

6 double unders, 5 push-ups

5 double unders, 6 push-ups

4 double unders, 7 push-ups

3 double unders, 8 push-ups

2 double unders, 9 push-ups

1 double under, 10 push-ups

REST FOR 2 MINUTES

1 double under, 10 push-ups

2 double unders, 9 push ups

3 double unders, 8 push-ups

4 double unders, 7 push-ups

5 double unders, 6 push-ups

6 double unders, 5 push-ups

7 double unders, 4 push-ups

8 double unders, 3 push-ups

9 double unders, 2 push-ups

10 double unders, 1 push-up

*Only rest at the halfway mark as instructed (for 2 minutes).

NOTES: This is a tough one, set a nice consistent pace and try to hold it the entire time.

(8) Perform 4 sets of the following:

-Max jump rope

-Max plank

-Max double unders

*Rest 2 minutes between exercises and 5 minutes between sets.

NOTES: Max means that you perform as many reps as you can before failure. In the case of plank you simply hold the plank position for as long as you possibly can before quitting. Once you fail, the exercise is over and the rest period begins. See how consistent you can be in your exercise reps. Push yourself to the limit on this workout!

(9) 6 Sets of the following:

1:00 speed skipping

10 squat jumps

30 seconds double unders

20 mountain climbers

1:00 speed skipping

30 seconds double unders

* Rest 30 seconds between exercises and 1:30 between sets.

(10) Perform 3 sets of the following:

150 jump rope

25 single leg skip (left)

25 single leg skip (right)

25 double unders

90 second plank

20 push ups 5 burpees

25 crossovers

25 jumping jack skipping

25 ski skipping

25 speed skipping

* Rest 20 seconds between exercises and 2 minutes between sets.

(1) 3 X 5 minutes unbroken jump rope.

*Rest 4 minutes between sets.

NOTES: If you mess up at all during any of the 5-minute sets you must restart that set with no rest. This doesn't mean that you have to restart the entire workout, but just the set you're currently on. The key to this workout is to develop a good pace that you can hold for 5 whole minutes. This workout isn't really too bad if you get it on the first try, but if you continue to make mistakes it will prove to be very difficult.

(2) 8 sets of the following:

40 double unders

15 push-ups

20 mountain climbers

10 burpees

*Rest 15 seconds between exercises and 2 minutes between sets.

(3) Complete the following as fast as possible:

3:00 double unders

6:00 freestyle skipping

10:00 plank

8:00 wall sit

2:00 burpees.

*Rest as needed.

NOTES: The total exercise time for this workout is 28 minutes. This can be split up however you like by taking chunks out of each exercise time. For example, you could do 30 seconds of double unders, 2:00 of freestyle skipping, 2:00 plank, 1:00 wall sit, etc. Just make sure you're keeping track of how long you're doing each exercise so you can ensure that you're not doing too much or too little. You can do the exercises in any order that you want.

(4) Perform 3 sets of the following:

1:00 jump rope

1:00 boxing jump rope

1:00 crossovers

1:00 ski skipping

1:00 jumping jack skipping

1:00 single leg skipping (right)

1:00 single leg skipping (left)

30 seconds double unders

30 seconds heel skipping

*Rest 30 seconds between exercises and 3 minutes between sets.

(5) 6 sets of 20 seconds on, 20 seconds off of the following exercises:

- Squat jumps
- Mountain climbers

- Double unders
- Push-ups
- Speed skipping
- Burpees

*Rest only 20 seconds between exercises and 1:30 between sets.

NOTES: This workout should be done at maximum intensity.

(6) 5 X 25 reps of the following exercises:

- Speed skaters
- Lunge walks
- Double unders
- Seal jacks
- Speed skipping
- Squat jumps

*Rest 30 seconds between exercises and 2 minutes between sets.

(7) Perform 4 sets of 30 seconds of each exercise:

- Heel skipping
- Double under crossovers
- Ski skipping
- Jumping jack skipping
- Boxing jump rope
- Double unders

*Rest 15 seconds between exercises and 2 minutes between sets.

THEN: perform jump rope for as long as you can until failure.

NOTES: The final part of the workout (max duration jump rope) isn't part of the main set and should only be done once the workout has been completed. Time yourself on this and try to see how long you can go for.

(8) You have 20 minutes to gain as many points as possible. Each exercise corresponds to a point value; the harder the exercise, the more it's worth. This workout is best done with a partner or a group so that you can compete to see who can gain the most points in the 20 minute time period.

Speed skipping- 1 PT

Seal jacks- 1 PT

Mountain Climbers- 2 PTS

Reverse crunches- 2 PTS

Push-ups- 3 PTS

Squat jumps- 3 PTS

Double unders- 3 PTS

Double under crossovers- 4 PTS

Burpees- 4 PTS

*Rest as needed, but remember you need to get as many points as possible so rest responsibly!

NOTES: Try to ensure that even when you're resting you're gathering some points by doing seal jacks or speed skipping.

(9) Perform 1 set of the following:

60 double unders, 60 seal jacks

50 double unders, 50 jumping jacks

40 double unders, 40 reverse crunches

30 double unders, 30 mountain climbers

20 double unders, 20 push-ups

10 double unders, 10 burpees

10 double unders, 10 burpees

20 double unders, 20 push-ups

30 double unders, 30 mountain climbers

40 double unders, 40 reverse crunches

50 double unders, 50 jumping jacks

60 double unders, 60 seal jacks

*Rest 30 seconds between every exercise and 2 minutes after reaching the halfway mark (upon completing the first set of 10 double unders and 10 burpees).

NOTES: This workout obviously requires a ton of double unders so make sure you're well warmed up!

(10) In 15 minutes complete as many sets as possible of the following sequence:

20 speed skipping

10 double unders

5 burpees

10 lunge walks

5 squat jumps

*Rest when needed.

I am a firm believer in not having to go to the gym to live a healthy and fit life. I would be lying if I told you that I didn't enjoy going to the gym on occasion, but the fact of the matter is: **a gym is not a prerequisite for fitness! Hard work, motivation, detailed planning and persistence are the only things that will get you fit.** The best part about these 4 aspects of fitness is that they can be done at home!

I really hope you try every workout in this book over the next 30 days. Keep in mind that if you're finding the workouts too easy or too difficult you can always tamper with the set numbers or the exercise repetitions/ times so that they suit you better. This book is by no means supposed to serve as a workout plan that has been chiseled in stone. Since I do not know you personally it makes it very difficult to create a workout plan for you, which is why I've included beginner, intermediate and advanced workouts in this book. Someday in the near future I plan to start an online personal training business, and then it will become much easier to help people achieve their personal fitness goals by creating workouts that are catered to their exact needs.

If you liked this book then I suggest that you check out some of my other fitness titles. Here's a sample of one of my top books on the next page, enjoy!

"Being halfway in anything is always the hardest part. But once you take one step past halfway, it's all downhill!"

- John Mayo

How To Get Abs: 2-in-1 Flat Stomach Boxed Set

How to Get Abs Fast With An Extensive 6-Week Workout Plan

John Mayo

© 2015

Copyright/ Disclaimer Information

This book is not intended as a substitute for the medical advice of physicians. The reader should regularly consult a physician in matters relating to his/her health and particularly with respect to any symptoms that may require diagnosis or medical attention.

Table of Contents:

1) Introduction:

If you don't have to work hard for something, then it's usually not worth getting!

We all know why you're here, so let's get right down to it. First things first, congratulations for taking it upon yourself to flatten out your stomach. Abs and a flat stomach are probably the most desired aspect of the human body for a lot of people. Human beings will put themselves through immense pain at the gym, just so they can feel good about themselves when they take off their shirts. Can you really blame these people though? Let's face it; abs and a flat stomach look great and it's completely understandable that people want to achieve this look.

So who am I and why should you care? I'm the guy who's going to help you achieve your fitness goals. I'm a guy who has had abs for almost his entire life. I'm not being cocky about it; it's just a fact. I have been an athlete for my entire life and fitness is something that I take very seriously. I am a kayaking coach in Nova Scotia, Canada, and my passion is helping people increase their fitness level. Since abs are a very sought after thing, I really enjoy helping people flatten their stomachs and get ripped abs.

Let me be honest though, abs are not easy to get, nor are they easy to maintain. Anything in life that is worthwhile takes hard work and dedication to achieve and getting abs is no different. I have a theory about abs; I think that one of the main things that make abs so sexy is that when people see a flat stomach or ripped abs, they understand the hard work and self-discipline associated with this achievement. I think a lot of people view a person's stomach as a direct reflection of their personality, so when somebody has no belly fat, people generally think of that person as dedicated, focused and determined. Unless of course they cheated and got liposuction. Perhaps you think this theory is a stretch, but I believe it to hold quite true for most people.

So what makes this fitness book different from all the other "get abs fast" books out there? One word, honesty. I will not lie to you and tell you that at the end of this 6-week program you will have the chiseled abs and flat stomach that you've always desired. But if you take the information, workout techniques and fitness strategies that I am going to provide to you in the following pages, apply them continuously and never give up, you will undoubtedly get the results that you desire.

Make no mistake; this is going to be a difficult task. I talk a lot in my other fitness books about forming good habits. One you make something a habit, it becomes automatic and easy. The less you have to think about making good, healthy choices, the better off your life will be. This is why it is very important to get into good fitness routines and stick with them! That's where I come in. I am very good at getting people into healthy routines and creating manageable programs that will better their health. This specific book is obviously going to focus on how to get abs and if you follow along and do not stray from my program, I can almost guarantee that you will see results. Strap yourselves in, focus, tighten those abs up and let's get going!

2) Abs Behind the Scenes:

If you're going to ignore your eating habits completely and strictly focus on exercise, don't bother reading any further. Contrary to popular belief, diet is the MOST important factor for getting abs. It doesn't matter how many fantastic abdominal exercises you do everyday, if you're eating fatty, deep fried, over-processed foods, you're not going to see results.

-What I Try to Avoid:

Fried foods, white rice, bread, potatoes, cereal, beer/ liquid carbs, fatty sauces, trans fats (obviously), high fructose corn syrup (glucose- fructose in Canada).

* I consume every single thing listed above; I just try to consume very minimal amounts of each.

-What I Typically Try to Eat:

Quinoa & quinoa pasta, whole grain or multigrain bread (if I eat bread at all), avocadoes, kale, spinach, max 2-3 eggs a day, brown rice, ground flaxseed (frozen or refrigerated), chia seeds (great mixed with water), chicken breast, ground tomatoes (substitute for pasta sauce), bananas, natural peanut/ almond butter, dates, unsalted nuts and almonds, black beans, cliff bars, mixed vegetables, unsweetened almond milk, unsweetened coconut water/ oil, LOTS AND LOTS OF WATER!

If you only allow healthy food in your living space, it will make things a lot easier when you have a craving for something bad. Here are some meals you could make that I really enjoy:

Breakfast:

1) Large smoothie consisting of 1 banana, 4 dates, 1 tbs of natural peanut butter, 1 handful or kale/ spinach, 1 tbs of ground flaxseed, 1 tbs of chia seeds, 1 tbs of coconut oil, 1 teaspoon of honey, lots of cinnamon, 1 handful of assorted frozen fruit, unsweetened almond milk and coconut water (add until there's a sufficient amount of liquid in the smoothie.)

2) 2 eggs and two pieces of toast. On the toast I like to put natural peanut butter, a little bit of honey and cinnamon.

3) Egg banana pancakes. 1 banana blended up with two eggs. Make just like you would pancakes. I like to add cinnamon and a touch of maple syrup.

Lunch:

1) Kale & spinach salad. Add avocado, chickpeas, ground flaxseed and black beans. For dressing I like to use a tiny bit of balsamic vinegar.

2) Pan fried haddock and a sweet potato with coconut oil.

3) Tuna sandwich on rye or flaxseed bread. I like to add lettuce, tomato and a bit of siracha sauce or pesto.

Dinner:

1) Spaghetti squash cooked in the oven. I like to add crushed tomatoes or a little bit of pesto.

2) Mango avocado salad. I use one mango and avocado, cut them up and add black beans, lettuce, jalapeños, quinoa, salsa and low fat corn chips. My personal favorite.

3) Mini pita pizzas. Add some pesto to pita bread with tomatoes, red pepper, onions and cheese. Bake the pita by the oven by itself first, add everything else and then put it back in the oven until the cheese melts.

The point I'm trying to make is that you need to take responsibility for your own diet. Keep in mind that diets should not be temporary. Your diet should be your lifestyle; you should make eating well a lifelong habit instead of a two-week fad. Temporary diets often lead to massive relapses in unhealthy eating. Lots of people start themselves out on unrealistic diets and never allow themselves to take a 'cheat day' and indulge in some tasty treats every once in a while. If you don't take a cheat day (I recommend once a week) you're sure to burn out and fail at your dieting plan.

Focus on your diet even harder than you focus on your exercises. If you get noting else out of this book please remember that no amount of abdominal exercise will get you a six pack/ flat stomach if you are eating like crap. Make no mistake, you will be strengthening your abs and getting a six pack if you eat like crap and workout like crazy, but I don't see much of a point in having abs if your stomach fat is covering it up. Your diet/ eating habits are key and you must not forget that!

Printed in Great Britain
by Amazon